1

Radiant Revitalization

The Collagen Diet for

Women

Unlocking Beauty, Health, and Vitality through Nourishing Collagen-Infused

Nutrition

2

3

Table of contents

4

4

5

n

5

Description

Do you want to have more energy, look younger, and feel more resilient?

Would you like to nourish your body from the inside out with the most common protein in your body? Are you curious about which foods and supplements wil increase the amount of col agen your body produces and prevent it from deteriorating?

If you can answer any of these questions, this book is for you. Col agen is a vital protein that gives your skin, bones, joints, muscles, and hair structure and suppleness. It also promotes wound healing, cel ular communication, and immune system function. As you become older, your body produces less col agen, which can lead to a variety of aging symptoms like wrinkles, sagging skin, joint pain, and hair loss.

You are not, however, required to take these modifications for granted. You can reverse or at least slow down the aging process with a diet high in col agen. With this book, you wil learn:

6

What col agen is, how important it is for your overal health and attractiveness, and how to eat more foods high in col agen, like dairy, fish, chickcn, cggs, and bonc broth

- How to choose the col agen supplements based on your needs and preferences

- How to avoid diets and lifestyle choices that accelerate aging and break down col agen

- How to prepare delicious, easy-to-make meals that wil boost col agen for breakfast, lunch, dinner, and snacks.

. How to assess your growth and see how it affects your skin, nails, hair, and body

Fol owing the col agen diet for women can improve your overal health and wel -being as wel as your appearance. You'l be happier, more energetic, and more confident. Furthermore, you wil identify, manage, and avoid a variety of prevalent health issues such as inflammation, leaky gut, osteoporosis, and arthritis.

Do not postpone any longer. You could see the difference in a matter of weeks if you start your col agen journey now. Get a copy of the Col agen Diet for Women today and get ready to shine!

7

Introduction

Have you ever wondered why your skin seems radiant, your hair shines, and your bones are sturdy? The solution lies in col agen, the most abundant protein in your body and the secret to both health and beauty.

Col agen makes up the majority of the connective tissues in your body, which include your skin, bones, cartilage, tendons, ligaments, and blood vessels. It supports metabolism, immunological response, wound healing, and the elasticity, sturdiness, and hydration of your tissues.

But as you age, your skin loses both quantity and quality of col agen.

Wrinkles, sagging skin, brittle nails, dryness, dul ness, thinning hair, joint pain, stiffness, inflammation, osteoporosis, poor wound healing, increased risk of infection, decreased muscle mass, strength, slowed metabolism, and weight gain are some of the symptoms associated with aging.

The good news is that you can halt or even reverse col agen loss with a col agen diet, or eating pattern that boosts col agen levels and provides extra health and cosmetic benefits. A col agen diet includes col agen-rich foods like bone broth, skin-on chicken, pork bone broth, sardines, oysters,

eggs, soy, spirulina, and col agen peptides, as wel as foods that protect and encourage col agen synthesis, such as fruits, vegetables, nuts, seeds, whole grains, and antioxidants. Supplementing with col agen or consuming col agen-boosting foods, beverages, and advice on a regular basis are other components of a col agen diet.

This book contains al the knowledge you need to understand col agen and how it affects the body. Discover the many uses for col agen, its various forms, the causes and warning signs of col agen depletion, how to prevent it, what foods are highest in col agen and how to cook them, the benefits and drawbacks of col agen supplements, and how to choose the best one for you. These are delicious and easy col agen-boosting recipes that you can make at home or on the go.

I developed this book because I have experienced firsthand the amazing benefits of col agen for both appearance and health. I used to suffer joint issues, dry, dul , and sagging skin, brittle nails, thinning hair, and poor energy. I tried a lot of products and treatments, but nothing seemed to help.

I decided to test col agen after knowing more about it. I started taking col agen pil s, eating more foods high in col agen, and fol owing some tips

9

on how to increase col agen in my body. In a short of weeks, I noticed a noticeable change in both my appearance and general health. My mood and energy increased, my skin became more luminous, firm, and moisturized, my hair grew thicker and shinier, my nails became stronger and healthier, and my joints felt more flexible and comfy. I received lots of praise from my friends, family, and coworkers, and I felt like a completely different person.

If you want to achieve the same results and enhance your beauty and health, this book is for you. If you fol ow the col agen diet, you wil feel better and look younger and more appealing. You'l be amazed at the results and wonder why you didn't start sooner. So why do you wait? Grab a copy of this book and begin your col agen journey right now. You deserve it!

10

Chapter 1

What Collagen Is All About

The structural backbone of our bodies, col agen is not your typical protein; it is the thread that runs through our nails, skin, hair, and connective tissues. Think of it as nature's scaffolding, supporting and giving the human form's complicated design structure.

Col agen is fundamental y a fibrous protein with an amazing molecular structure. Imagine a web of interwoven chains that forms a sturdy structure and provides our tissues with their elasticity and strength. This molecular wonder is the foundation of col agen, providing the structural integrity that characterizes our physical existence.

Comprehending the nature of col agen entails more than just acknowledging it as an element; it involves realizing its function as an essential constituent. Imagine col agen as the quiet architect that shapes our bodies' form and function in subtle yet crucial ways as we set out on this trip. We wil work together to solve the secrets of this remarkable protein and discover how its fundamentals fit into the overal picture of human wel -being and attractiveness.

11

How Important It Is for Women

1.Women's unique Health Considerations.

Women travel through several stages that are distinguished by changes in hormones and particular health issues. This section explores the complex interactions between these variables and col agen, highlighting the critical role that it plays at various points in a woman's life.

Col agen joins young girls as they enter the dance of hormonal shifts as they develop femininity. Establishing a foundation of holistic health requires an understanding of this connection. We examine how col agen changes to support women's particular physiological needs, from youth's resiliency to maturity's wisdom.

2. Beauty Beyond Aesthetics

Women benefit from col agen in ways that go beyond cosmetics. Beyond the search for outward beauty, we set out on a scientific investigation to learn more about its significant influence. Col agen serves as a potent al y in maintaining a young appearance by enhancing glowing skin and minimizing the visible signs of aging.

12

By deciphering the science underlying col agen's ability to enhance beauty, we enable women to adopt a holistic perspective on their health. The importance is in fostering the body's natural capacity to exude health from the inside out, not only in terms of appearance.

Join us on this voyage of discovery as we honor the complex role that col agen plays in women's lives, a trip that encompasses health, vitality, and the ageless beauty that results from an internal harmony.

3. Connecting Science to Daily Life

• Linking Theory and Practice

This is a crucial area where we help you make the transition from scientific understanding to real-world application by walking you through the process of integrating col agen into your daily routine. We go from knowing the theoretical underpinnings to practical measures that enable you to take advantage of col agen's benefits.

Set off on a gastronomic adventure as we explore a variety of col agen-rich food sources. We reveal the range of options that can increase your consumption of col agen, from enjoying nutrient-dense bone broth to

13

including foods high in col agen into your meals. It's not only about knowing what to do; it's also about applying your knowledge to make decisions that fit your way of life.

● Lifestyle Decisions to Increase Col agen.

Beyond the plate, col agen optimization is greatly influenced by lifestyle decisions. We reveal the techniques of skincare regimens that go below the surface in this episode. Develop routines that protect against the elements that lead to the deterioration of col agen while simultaneously promoting its production.

We explore the art of holistic wel -being, covering everything from protecting your skin from the sun's rays to forming routines that encourage the synthesis of col agen. This is a conscious approach to everyday decisions that enhance the benefits of col agen, not a regimen. Enhancing your col agen journey is not only a science; it's an art, created on the canvas of your daily rituals, as we weave the connections between science and your everyday life.

Come explore in a way that puts theory into practice and shows you how the deep science of col agen can be woven into every aspect of your daily life. It's not just about knowing; it's about living your life to the ful est and al owing col agen's transformational power to flow with your own rhythm.

14

Chapter 2

Interpreting Diversity in Collagen and Its Effects on Your Body

This chapter wil enlighten you on the numerous forms of col agen and how they affect your body. Welcome to the discovery of the complex tapestry of col agen.

1: Variety of Col agen

A protein cal ed col agen gives your body's tissues and organs strength, support, and structure. Col agen comes in various forms, each with unique properties and uses. The primary forms of col agen and their effects on your body are outlined below:

• Type I col agen makes up about 90% of the col agen found in the body, this gives your skin, bones, tendons, and ligaments structure.

It's also present in your hair, placenta, and cornea.

15

• Type 11 col agen contains elastic cartilage, which supports and cushions your ears and nose. cartilage, the pliable tissue that lies between bones, is made possible by it.

• Col agen type III is present in your arteries, muscles, and organs. It aids in the development of blood vessels and muscles. Additional y, it maintains the suppleness and structure of your skin.

• Type IV Col agen can be found in the layers of your skin, particularly in the basement membrane that divides the outer layer (epidermis) from the middle layer (dermis). It supports cel development and aids in substance filtering.

• Type V col agen is found on the cornea of your eyes, some skin layers, hair, and placental tissue . It aids in the formation of type I col agen fibrils and type IV col agen networks.

16

symptoms and causes of collagen loss, How to Prevent or Reverse it.

The fol owing are the symptoms, causes, and preventative/reversal measures for col agen loss:

Signs

The fol owing are some typical indications of col agen loss 1.A decrease in the face's natural ful ness, particularly in the cheek and under-eye areas

2.Reduced flexibility and cushioning of cartilage causes degeneration and joint pains.

3.Sagging skin, particularly around the stomach, butt, and jawline. Wrinkles and fine lines, particularly around the mouth, forehead, and eyes.

4.Unhealthy hair and hair loss lead to thin, brittle, and dul hair.

17

Causes

1.Sun exposure, which damages col agen fibers and speeds up the aging process of the skin.

2.Aging, which natural y lowers the body's production and quality of col agen.

3. Environmental pol utants, such as smoke, dust, and chemicals, which can cause oxidative stress and inflammation that degrade col agen **Prevention and reversal**

Some strategies to stop or reverse col agen loss include: 1.Eating a wel -balanced diet that contains adequate protein, vitamin C, zinc, copper, and manganese—nutrients crucial for col agen production.

Poor diet can deprive the body of the essential amino acids, vitamins, and minerals needed to synthesize col agen. Animal skin and bones, bone broth, eggs, fish, poultry, meat, dairy products, citrus fruits, berries, leafy greens, nuts, and seeds are a few foods high in col agen.

2.Consuming col agen supplements, including hydrolyzed col agen or col agen peptides, which the body can absorb and use with ease12.

18

3. Preventing sun damage to the skin by wearing hats, sunglasses, sunscreen, and clothing that covers exposed areas. - Refraining from smoking, drinking alcohol, and consuming sugar, as these activities can reduce col agen synthesis and increase its breakdown.

4.Using topical products that contain ingredients that boost col agen, such as retinoids, vitamin C, peptides, and antioxidants, which can boost col agen production and shield the skin from free radicals.

19

Chapter 3

The best Foods High in Collagen and How to Make Them

1. Bone Broth: Supercharged with nutrients: In addition to being high in col agen, bone broth contains amino acids including proline and glycine, which are essential for the synthesis of col agen.Col agen type I, which is beneficial to your skin, hair, and nails, is abundant in bone broth.

Preparation:Simmer a mixture of bones (chicken, beef, hog, or fish), veggies, and seasonings to make a fil ing bone broth. Enjoy it on its own for a nutrient boost, or use it as a base for stews and soups.

2. Avocado:Healthy Fats:The monounsaturated fats in avocados enhance the moisture and flexibility of the skin, enhancing the advantages of col agen.

Preparation

Eat avocado sliced on whole-grain toast, pureed into smoothies for a healthy and fil ing snack, or added to salads for smoothness.

20

3.Chicken: Another good source of type I col agen is chicken, particularly in the skin and cartilage. Skin-on chicken is edible, and bone broth can be made from the bones and feet of the bird. Additional y rich in protein, chicken encourages your body to create more col agen.

Preparation

Prepare the chicken by roasting, gril ing, baking, or stir-frying it with your preferred vegetables and seasonings. With leftover chicken, you may also prepare salads, sandwiches, and chicken soup.

4. Seafoods: Rich in col agen type II, fish and shel fish are beneficial to your cartilage and joints. Omega-3 fatty acids, which have anti-inflammatory and skin-protective properties, are also found in seafood.

Seafood is available to eat raw, cooked, or canned. Seafood such as shrimp, oysters, scal ops, sardines, mackerel, tuna, and salmon are some of the richest sources of col agen. Seafood is a great addition to salads, sandwiches, soups, curries, and sushi.

Preparation

Toss fish on the gril or bake it with lemon, herbs, and olive oil for a tasty and col agen-boosting main dish.

21

5. Egg whites: Rich in protein, egg whites include a lot of proline and glycine, two amino acids that are necessary for the formation of col agen.

Sulfur is another ingredient found in egg whites that helps stop col agen deterioration.

Preparation

Egg whites can be poached, fried, scrambled, or boiled. Egg whites can also be used to make meringues, frittatas, quiches, and omelets.

6. Citrus fruits: Rich in vitamin C, a cofactor for the synthesis of col agen, citrus fruits include oranges, grapefruits, lemons, and limes. Additional y, vitamin C helps shield your skin from free radicals and the sun, which can weaken col agen.

Preparation

Citrus fruits can be consumed fresh, juiced, or dried. Additional y, you can flavor salads, marinades, sauces, desserts, and dressings using citrus zest or juice.

7. Berries: Rich in antioxidants and vitamin C, berries like strawberries, blueberries, raspberries, and blackberries help to protect and produce

22

col agen. Additional y, berries include el agic acid, which may help to reduce inflammation and the deterioration of col agen.

Preparation

Berries can be consumed frozen, dried, or fresh. Berries can also be added to baked products, cereal, yogurt, oatmeal, and smoothies.

8. Tropical foods: Rich in vitamin C and other antioxidants, tropical fruits like pineapple, mango, papaya, and kiwi promote the creation of col agen and the health of the skin. Enzymes found in tropical fruits, notably papain and bromelain, may aid in the digestion of col agen and other proteins.

Preparation

Tropical fruits can be consumed fresh, frozen, or dried. Tropical fruits can also be added to salads, desserts, salsas, and smoothies.

9. Garlic: Sulfur is abundant in garlic and is essential for the production of col agen and cross-linking. Al icin, another ingredient in garlic, may shield col agen from deterioration and aging.

Preparation

Garlic can be consumed fresh, cooked, or powdered. Garlic can also be added to roasts, stir-fries, dips, soups, and sauces.

23

10. Leafy greens: Rich in chlorophyl , leafy greens including spinach, kale, col ard greens, and Swiss chard may boost procol

agen, the precursor to col agen, in your skin. In addition, leafy greens are rich in antioxidants, vitamin C, and vitamin A, al of which promote the formation and maintenance of col agen.

Preparation

Leafy greens can be prepared in one of three ways: cooked, raw, or blended. Leafy greens can also be added to wraps, smoothies, soups, and salads.

Sauté with olive oil and garlic to make a tasty side dish.

11. Beans: Rich in protein, which supplies the amino acids needed for the formation of col agen, beans include kidney beans, chickpeas, black beans, and soybeans. Copper, another nutrient found in beans, is necessary for the synthesis of col agen and cross-linking.

Preparation

Beans can be consumed, cooked, tinned, or sprouted. Beans can also be added to dips, stews, soups, and salads.

24

12. Cashews: Rich in copper, zinc, and iron, al essential for the synthesis and upkeep of col agen. Cashews are a great source of these minerals.

Additional y rich in protein, antioxidants, and good fats, cashews promote the suppleness and health of the skin.

Preparation

Cashews can be eaten buttered, roasted, or raw. Cashews can also be added to curries, salads, stir-fries, and desserts.

13. Tomatoes: Rich in lycopene, a potent antioxidant that shields your skin against UV rays and the deterioration of col agen,

tomatoes are a great source of antioxidants. Vitamin C, which aids in the formation of col agen, is also present in tomatoes.

Preparation

Tomatoes can be eaten canned, cooked, or fresh. Tomatoes can also be added to pizzas, salads, sandwiches, soups, and sauces.

14. Bel peppers: Rich in vitamin C and carotenoids, which are antioxidants that improve skin health and col agen formation, bel peppers, especial y red ones, are a great source of vitamin C. Additional y present in bel

25

peppers is capsaicin, which has been shown to enhance skin tone and blood flow.

Preparation

Bel peppers can be eaten fresh, sautéed, or roasted. Bel peppers can also be added to stuffed peppers, fajitas, stir-fries, and salads.

26

Chapter 4

Collagen Supplements: Their Advantages and Disadvantages and How to Pick the Best One for You

Supplements containing col agen sourced from plants or animals are known as col agen supplements. The structure and health of your skin, bones, joints, muscles, and other tissues depend on the protein col agen.

Supplemental col agen is touted for its ability to improve skin suppleness, minimize wrinkles, ease joint discomfort, and strengthen bones, among other things. But not every col agen supplement is made equal, and some can have disadvantages or restrictions. Here are some advantages and disadvantages of col agen supplements, along with advice on which one is best for you.

27

Collagen supplement benefits

1. **Skin health**: Col agen supplements can help your skin become more hydrated, elastic, and dense while also reducing aging indicators like wrinkles and drooping. This is because taking col agen supplements may encourage your body to manufacture more col agen and other skin-related proteins like elastin and fibril in. (Col agen is a major component of your skin.)

2. **Joint health:** Especial y in patients with osteoarthritis or rheumatoid arthritis, col agen supplements may help lessen joint discomfort, stiffness, and inflammation. This is due to the fact that col agen plays a crucial role in the cartilage that protects and cushions your joints. By taking col agen supplements, you may be able to protect your cartilage and stop additional damage1.

3. **Bone health**: Especial y for postmenopausal women, col agen supplements may help increase bone growth, density, and strength. This is because taking col agen supplements may encourage your

body to manufacture more proteins associated with bones, such osteocalcin and osteopontin, as col agen makes up a significant portion of your bones.

28

4. **Muscle health:** Especial y for older folks or those suffering from sarcopenia (age-related muscle loss), col agen supplements may help you gain more muscle mass, strength, and performance. This is due to the fact that col agen makes up a large portion of your muscles, and taking col agen supplements may encourage your body to manufacture more proteins connected to muscles, such myosin and creatine.

5. **Heart health:** Supplementing with col agen may help lower blood pressure, cholesterol, and triglycerides while also enhancing the suppleness and function of your blood vessels. This is because taking col agen supplements may encourage your body to make more col agen and other vascular-related proteins like nitric oxide and endothelin.

Col agen is a major component of your blood vessels.

29

Cons of taking collagen supplements

Col agen supplements may have certain disadvantages or restrictions in addition to their possible advantages, such as: 1. Absence of regulation: The Food and Drug Administration (FDA) does not regulate col agen supplements, which implies that there may be significant variations in their efficacy, safety, and quality. Certain col agen supplements could have impurities that are harmful to your health, like pesticides, heavy metals, or bacteria. Additional y, the labels on some col agen supplements may be erroneous or deceptive, which can make it chal enging to evaluate goods or figure out the ideal dosage.

2. Lack of evidence: Despite the fact that certain studies have demonstrated the beneficial effects of col agen supplements on a

range of health outcomes, the available data is stil few and unreliable. Due to their smal size, short duration, or supplement industry sponsorship, the majority of the research run the risk of bias or confounding variables. Further extensive, long-term, and independent research is required to validate the advantages and security of col agen supplements.

30

3. Poor absorption: Supplements containing col agen are often hydrolyzed, which reduces the peptides to tiny pieces that are simpler to absorb and digest. Nevertheless, a portion of these peptides might stil be too big to pass through the intestinal barrier and reach the circulation, which could restrict their efficacy and bioavailability. Furthermore, the function and activity of some of these peptides may change as a result of degradation or modification by bacteria or enzymes in the gut.

4. Lack of specificity: Different forms of col agen, such as type I, II, III, IV, or V, which have various roles and functions in the body, may be included in col agen supplements. It is unclear, nonetheless, if ingesting a particular kind of col agen supplement would target a particular tissue or organ or if it wil be dispersed equal y throughout the body. Moreover, it is unclear if consuming col agen supplements wil encourage the body to produce more of the same kind of col agen or other similar proteins.

5. Incompatibility: Supplemental col agen may originate from plant or animal sources, which may differ from human col agen in terms of characteristics and outcomes. The bioactivity and compatibility of animal and human col agen may differ due to differences in their molecular

31

structures, immunogenicity, and amino acid compositions. Plant col agen might be a blend of proteins and polysaccharides that imitate some of the properties of actual col agen instead of the real thing.

6. Lack of necessity: While some people may already have adequate or ideal amounts of col agen and other associated proteins in their bodies, supplements may not be required for everyone. Furthermore, consuming a balanced diet that includes sufficient amounts of protein, vitamin C, zinc, copper, and other elements necessary for col agen synthesis may help some people raise their col agen levels. A few lifestyle choices, like quitting smoking, getting enough sun exposure, and managing your stress, may also help maintain and protect your col agen.

32

How to pick your ideal collagen supplement

Fol owing your decision to use col agen supplements, the fol owing advice wil help you select the best kind for you: 1. Speak with your doctor: It is always good to speak with your doctor before taking any supplements, particularly if you have any al ergies or are currently on any drugs. Your physician can advise you on the proper quantity and duration of col agen supplementation as wel as assist you establish whether they are safe and suited for you.

2. Read the label: It's critical to look for the fol owing details on the label when selecting a col agen supplement:

• The kind and source of col agen: Seek out the kind of col agen type I for skin, type II for joints, or type III for blood vessels that best suits your health objective. Additional y, search for the col agen's source, be it plant, animal, fish, poultry, or cow, and select the one that aligns with your values and tastes.

33

• The quantity and quality of col agen: Find the amount of col agen per serving, which is typical y stated in mil igrams or grams, and select the quantity that meets your requirements. Additional y, find the col agen's purity, which is typical y indicated as a percentage, and select the col agen with the highest purity.

• substances and additives: Check for sweeteners, flavors, colors, preservatives, and fil ers among other substances in the col agen supplement, then select the one with the fewest artificial or superfluous ingredients. Additional y, check the col agen supplement for any potential al ergens or contaminants (including metals, dairy, gluten, or soy) and stay away from those that could result in negative reactions or pose a health risk.

• The certification and verification: Seek out certifications and verifications that attest to the safety and quality of the col agen supplement, such as United States Pharmacopeia (USP), Good Manufacturing Practices (GMP), or third-party testing, and select the most trustworthy and credible one.

3. Evaluate the cost and value: It's crucial to weigh the costs and benefits of several col agen supplements before making a decision. The cost per

34

gram or mil igram of col agen can be calculated by dividing the price by the amount of col agen per serving. Subsequently, you can evaluate the price per mil igram or gram of col agen in several goods and select the one that provides the most value for your money. When making your ultimate choice, you should, however, also take your satisfaction and personal preferences into account in addition to the col agen supplement's efficacy and quality.

35

Chapter 5

Collagen boosting Recipes, tips, and Tricks to increase Collagen in Your Daily Routine Try some of these methods and tricks to include col agen into your daily routine if you want to increase your col agen levels and reap the benefits of better skin, hair, nails, and joints:

1.Eat more foods high in col agen: A few foods that are high in col agen or that encourage your body to generate more of it are bone broth, chicken, shel fish, egg whites, citrus fruits, berries, tropical fruits, garlic, leafy greens, beans, cashews, tomatoes, and bel peppers.

2.Use a supplement containing col agen: Supplements containing col agen sourced from plants or animals are known as col agen supplements. In addition to providing several health advantages like increasing skin

36

elasticity, decreasing wrinkles, easing joint discomfort, and boosting bone health, they can aid in your body's col agen synthesis. But not every col agen supplement is made equal, and some can have disadvantages or restrictions.

3.Incorporate col agen into your beverages: Since col agen supplements are typical y sold in powder form, adding them to drinks is simple. Col agen powder can be combined with milk, juice, water, coffee, tea, or smoothies.

Flavored col agen powders, like SkinnyFit's Super Youth, can also be used to improve the flavor and nutritional value of your beverages.

4.Incorporate col agen into your baking and cooking: Since col agen powder dissolves readily and can tolerate high temperatures, it can also be utilized in baking and cooking. Col agen powder can be used in soups, sauces, dips, cakes, muffins, cookies, pancakes, waffles, and bread.

Col agen powder can also be used to make pudding, marshmal ows, and handmade gummies.

5.Apply col agen topical y: To help hydrate, nourish, and protect your skin, hair, and nails, col agen can also be applied topical y. Col agen-specific products such as oils, masks, serums, and creams can be applied topical y.

Additional y, you may create your own col agen beauty products at home

37

with natural components like essential oils, honey, coconut oil, and aloe vera.

Foods high in collagen

1. Chicken Thighs with Honey-Garlic w ith Broccoli and Carrots

This recipe for baked honey-garlic chicken thighs is sweet and flavorful, and it makes the ideal weekday supper with a side dish of vegetables that cook on the same sheet pan as the chicken.

Ingredients

1/4 cup honey

1 and a half tablespoons of tamari or reduced-sodium soy sauce four minced garlic cloves (approximately one and a half tablespoons) One tsp of apple cider vinegar

A tsp of finely ground red pepper

Eight five-ounce, skin-and-bone chicken thighs 1 pound of thinly sliced, half-inch-long carrots Two tsp olive oil, separated

4 cups (about 1 pound) of broccoli florets

38

Salt, ½ teaspoon

A smidgeon of ground pepper

One tsp cornstarch

one tsp water

Preparation

1. To prepare, combine honey, vinegar, crushed red pepper, garlic, soy sauce (or tamari), and a smal bowl. Put the chicken into a plastic bag with a zip-top and half of the honey mixture (about 1/4 cup); blot out any extra air and close the bag. Til the chicken is evenly coated, massage it within the closed bag. For a minimum of 30 minutes and a maximum of 2 hours, refrigerate. Keep the leftover combination of honey aside.

2. Turn the oven on to 400°F. Spread cooking spray on a large rimmed baking sheet and line it with foil. Take the chicken out of the marinade (throw away marinade); place on one side of the pan that has been preheated. In a medium-sized bowl, combine carrots and 1 tbsp oil; toss to coat. On the opposite side of the pan, evenly distribute the carrots. For fifteen minutes, bake the chicken and carrots. Take out of the oven and toss the carrots.

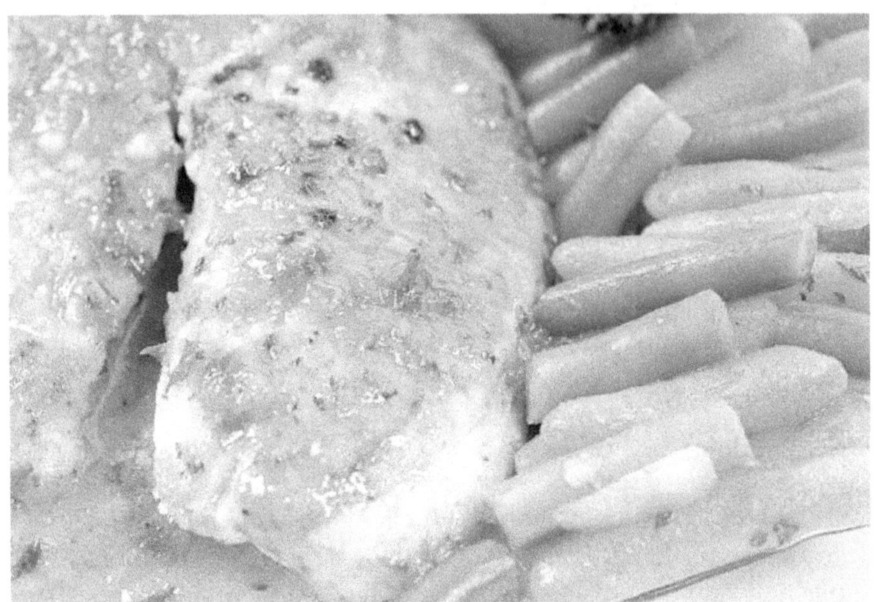

39

3. Mix the broccoli with the leftover 1 tablespoon of oil, making sure to thoroughly coat. Evenly scatter the broccoli atop the skil et of chicken and carrots. Season everything with salt & pepper. Bake for 15 to 18 minutes, or until the veggies are soft and a thermometer inserted into the thickest part of the chicken reads 165°F.

4. Meanwhile, in a smal dish, mix together cornstarch and water until no clumps remain. In a smal saucepan, combine the cornstarch mixture with the honey mixture that was set aside. Over medium-low heat, bring to a simmer while whisking once or twice. Simmer for about two minutes, stirring frequently, or until the sauce thickens and becomes clear. Pour some over the veggies and poultry. Warm up the food.

Chicken Thighs with Honey-Garlic w

ith Broccoli and Carrots

Equipment: large baking sheet with a rim To plan ahead: For up to four days, keep the marinade refrigerated in an airtight container.

40

2. Sardine Toasts with Peas and Fennel.

Upgrade plain toast with a verdant, vegetable-rich spread that includes sweet English peas, mint, and fennel. Two of these liberal y topped bruschetta-style toasts are wonderful as a light lunch with a salad, or one makes a great appetizer. Here, canned sardines and anchovies are excel ent, as wel as gril ed fresh sardines, if available.

Ingredients

Four whole-grain crackers in the Scandinavian style, including Wasa, Ry Krisp, Ryvita, and Kavli

8–12 sardines in cans, ideal y with olive oil packed in them 4 slices of lemon

Preparation

Place two or three sardines on top of each cracker. Add a squeeze of lemon for finishing.

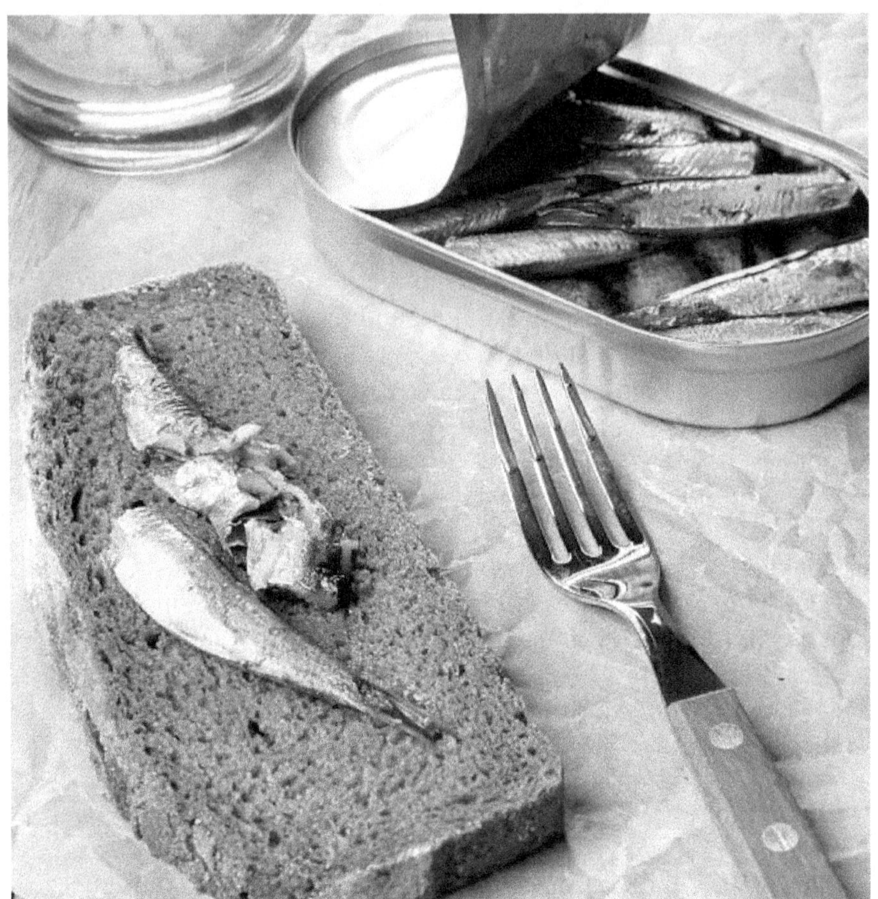

41

Sardine Toasts with Peas and Fennel

3. Broccoli with Balsamic and Parmesan Roasting.

Try this simple vegetable dish as an accompaniment to fish, poultry, or any other main course. It's delicious heated grain bowls or salads as wel .

Advice: Heating the pan beforehand promotes the nutty flavors and browning of the broccoli.

Ingredients

Eight cups of fresh broccoli (from two large heads) florets Three tsp olive oil

1 ½ ounces of grated Parmesan cheese (about 1/3 cup) One-half teaspoon of flaky sea salt, such Maldon, and two tablespoons of balsamic vinegar

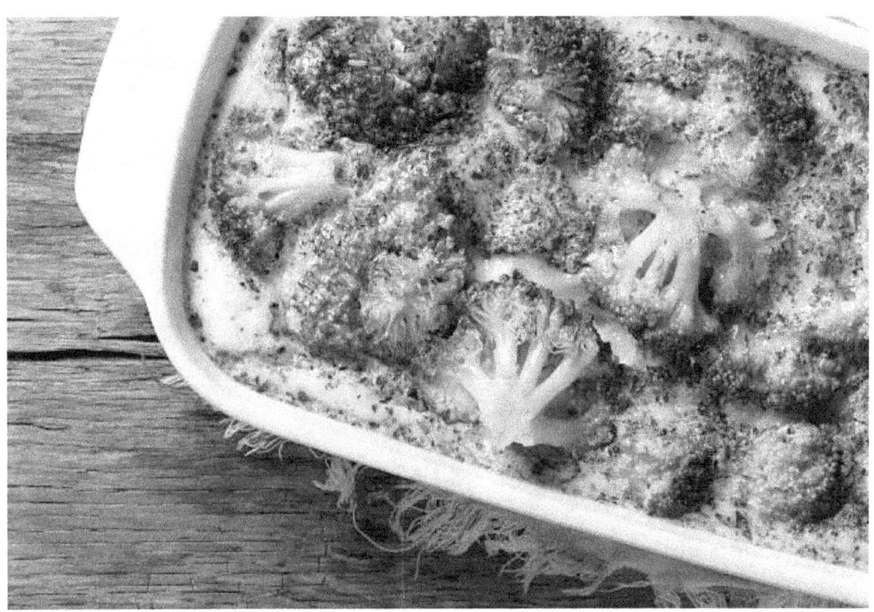

42

Preparation

1. Set the middle oven rack on the rimmed baking sheet, and preheat the oven to 425 degrees F. When the oven has finished preheating, leave the pan in there for five minutes.

2. In the meantime, put the broccoli in a big bowl with the oil and toss to coat. Arrange the broccoli on the heated baking sheet in a uniform layer.

Roast for about 17 minutes, or until beginning to brown. Take out of the oven and top with Parmesan cheese. Roast the broccoli for a further three to five minutes, or until it is soft and the cheese has melted. Serve right away after drizzling with vinegar and seasoning with salt.

Broccoli with Balsamic and Parmesan Roasting.

4. Fruit Salad with Strawberries

There's enough fruit salad for a crowd with this recipe for summer berries.

Serve with yogurt and granola for brunch, as a nutritious side dish for a potluck, or cut the recipe in half to serve 4.

Ingredients

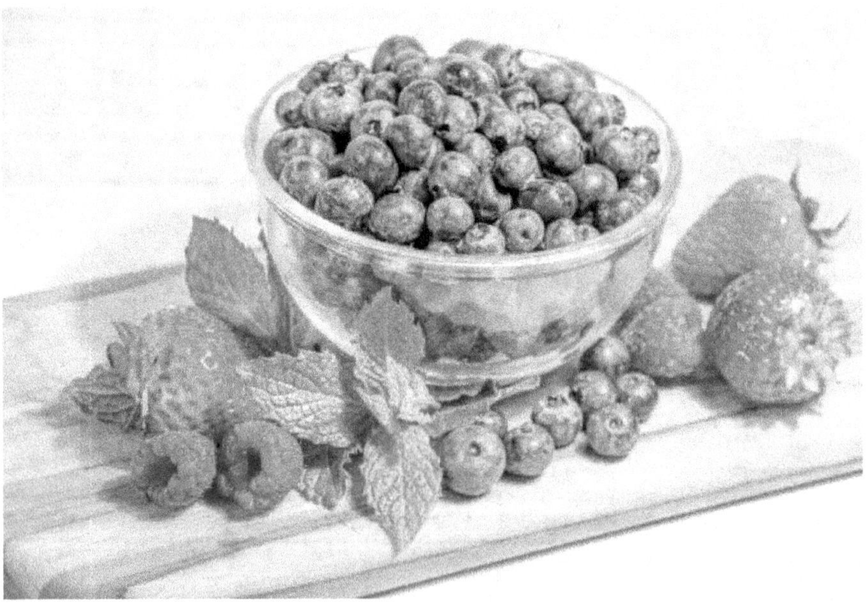

43

Two tsp of honey

two tsp of lemon juice

Six cups of fresh strawberries, hul ed and cut in half (or quarters, if huge) Double cups of raw blackberries

¼ cup of fresh mint, chopped finely

Preparation

In a big bowl, whisk together lemon juice and honey. Blackberries and strawberries should be added; toss gently to coat. Al ow to stand for thirty minutes or up to an hour. Add mint right before serving.

Fruit Salad with Strawberries

5. **Broccoli with Chicken in Herb Butter Sauce** Dinner with chicken and broccoli cooked in one skil et is flavorful, nutritious, and easy to prepare. We add a little stock and butter to the drippings after the chicken roasts to make a velvety, smooth pan sauce.

44

Ingredients

One tablespoon of pure olive oil

1-1/2 pounds of skin-on, bone-in chicken thighs ½ teaspoon of split kosher salt and ½ teaspoon of crushed pepper 4 cups florets of broccoli

4 ounces of shal ots, chopped, then cut in half lengthwise two minced garlic cloves

One teaspoon of freshly chopped sage, with extra for decoration 1 tsp finely chopped, recent rosemary

Two cups of stock, unsalted

two tsp of butter

Two cups warm, prepared brown rice

Preparation

1. Turn the oven on to 425°F.

2. In a big cast-iron skil et, heat the oil over medium-high heat.
Place the chicken skin-side down and cook for 6 to 10 minutes on
each side, or until golden, rotating once. After transferring,
sprinkle 1/2 teaspoon each of salt and pepper on both sides of the
dish.

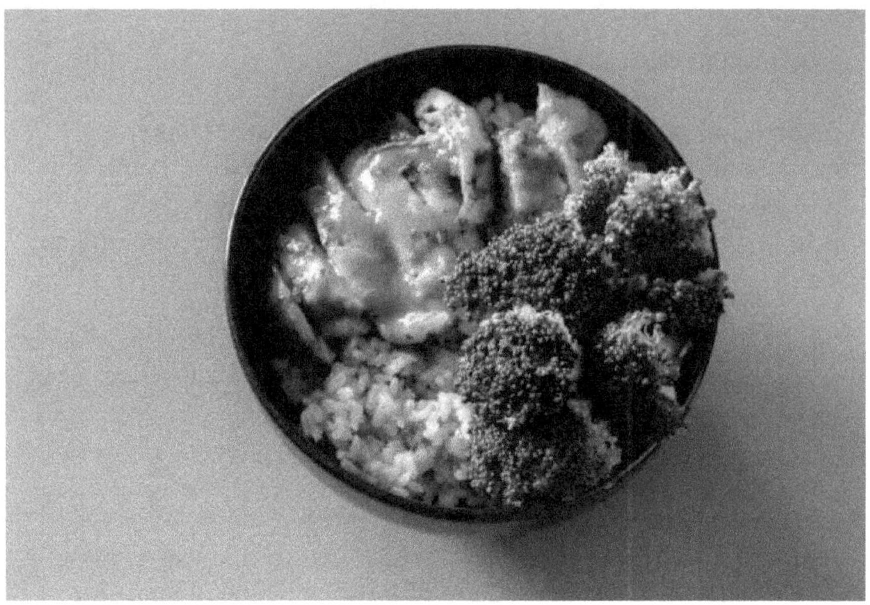

45

3.Toss the broccoli and shal ots in the pan to coat them in the pan
drippings. Stir in the garlic, sage, and rosemary and simmer for
one minute or until fragrant. Place the chicken in the oven,
nestling it on top of the veggies. Roast for about 8 minutes, or until
an instant-read thermometer placed into the thickest part of the
chicken, without touching the bone, reads 165°F.

4. Set the pan on medium-high heat, being cautious since the
handle wil get hot. Move the veggies and chicken to one side.
Simmer after adding the stock and scraping up any browned parts.
Add the butter and simmer for about 5 minutes, stirring often, or
until the sauce thickens. Add the final 1/4 teaspoon of salt on top.

Along with the rice, serve the chicken and veggies with the sauce.
If desired, garnish with more sage.

Broccoli with Chicken in Herb Butter Sauce **6. Garlic-Lemon
Sardine Fettuccine**

This citrusy pasta with crispy breadcrumbs is sure to wow even the
most skeptical sardine eaters. If you'd like, you may instead use
two 5- to 6-ounce cans of chunk light tuna in place of the sardines.
In St ep 4, along

46

with the lemon juice, add 2 teaspoons of tomato paste if you're
using tuna or can't find sardines wrapped in tomato sauce.
Accompany with a glass of Pinot Grigio and a salad of bitter
greens dressed with a lemon vinaigrette.

Ingredients

Whole-wheat fettuccine, 8 ounces

Four tsp extra virgin olive oil, split

four minced garlic cloves

One cup of freshly made breadcrumbs, preferably whole-wheat 1/4
cup of lemon juice

one tsp finely ground pepper

Salt, ½ teaspoon

Two three- to four-ounce cans of skinless, boneless sardines, best
served with tomato sauce, flakes

½ cup of freshly chopped parsley

Finely shred ¼ cup of Parmesan cheese

Preparation

1.Put a big saucepan of water on to the boil. Cook pasta according to package directions or until just cooked, 8 to 10 minutes. Empty.

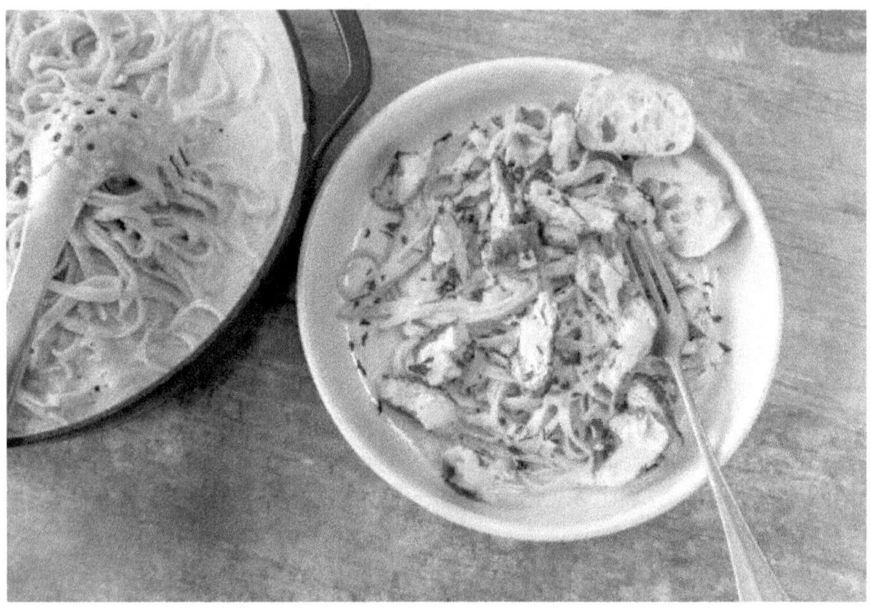

Garlic-Lemon Sardine Fettuccine

47

2. In the interim, place a smal nonstick skil et over medium heat with two teaspoons of oil. Add the garlic and heat, stirring, for approximately 20

seconds, or until it is fragrant and sizzling but not brown. Pour the oil and garlic into a big basin.

3. Place the pan's remaining two teaspoons of oil over medium heat. Stir in bread crumbs and heat for 5 to 6 minutes, or until golden brown and crispy.

Move to a platter.

4. Mix salt, pepper, and lemon juice with the garlic oil. Add the spaghetti, parsley, Parmesan, and sardines to the bowl. Stir gently to mix. Garnish with the breadcrumbs and serve.

Garlic-Lemon Sardine Fettuccine

Tips: Trim the crusts from whole-wheat bread in order to make fresh breadcrumbs. Break the bread into smal pieces and pulse it in a food processor to create coarse crumbs. A bread slice yields around half a cup of fresh crumbs.

48

8. **Salted Carrots with Roasted Chicken** A whole roasted chicken is the epitome of comfort food, but the cooking process can be lengthy. Instead, use the parts to make this simple roast chicken for a midweek meal. This Italian salsa verde sauce adds brightness with its fresh herbs, lemon juice, and capers.

Ingredients

One 4- to 5-pound entire chicken or four pounds of bone-in chicken parts Two tablespoons of extra virgin olive oil, four minced cloves of garlic, a ½

teaspoon each of kosher salt and powdered pepper, and two pounds of tiny carrots cut in half lengthwise are al divided.

One cup of finely chopped fresh herbs, like marjoram, basil, parsley, oregano,

two tsp of lemon juice

One tablespoon of washed capers

One tsp of pasted anchovies

One tablespoon of water

Preparation

1. Put two baking sheets with rims in the oven and warm it to 500 degrees.

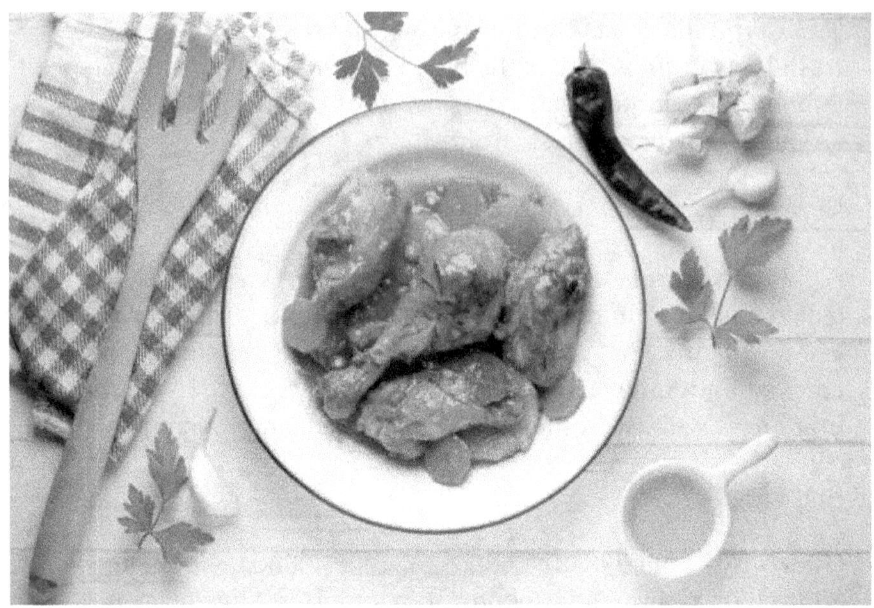

49

2. Cut the chicken into pieces if using a whole bird (breasts, leg quarters, and wings). Halve any chicken breasts lengthwise. In a smal bowl, mix together 1 tablespoon oil, half of the garlic, 1/2 teaspoon pepper, and salt.

Apply al over and under the skin of the bird.

3. After taking the pans out of the oven, split the chicken between them. On both pans, arrange carrots around the chicken.

4. Lower the oven's setting to 450 degrees. Cook the chicken and carrots for 20 to 30 minutes, or until an instant-read thermometer is put into the thickest portion of a leg and kept away from the bone registers 165 degrees Fahrenheit.

5. In the meantime, puree the remaining garlic, 1/4 teaspoon pepper, anchovy paste, lemon juice, capers, and herbs in a food processor. Pulse until chopped finely. Add the remaining 1 tablespoon of oil and the water gradual y while the motor is running.

6. Present the sauce alongside the chicken and carrots.

Salted Carrots with Roasted Chicken

50

9. **Banana, Blueberry, and Strawberry Smoothie** A smoothie made with banana, blueberries, and strawberries is mildly sweet and perfect for children, even with the added protein from hemp seeds. To achieve an extra-frosted texture after blending, freeze the fruits beforehand.

Ingredients

Half a cup of frozen strawberry

½ cup frozen blueberries

One little, ripe banana, frozen if preferred ¾ cup of chil ed cashew milk without sugar, or more if necessary One tsp cashew butter

One spoonful of hemp seeds, hul ed

Preparation

1. In a blender, combine hemp seeds, cashew milk, cashew butter, strawberries, blueberries, and banana. Blend until smooth, adding additional cashew milk as necessary to achieve the desired consistency.

Serve right away.

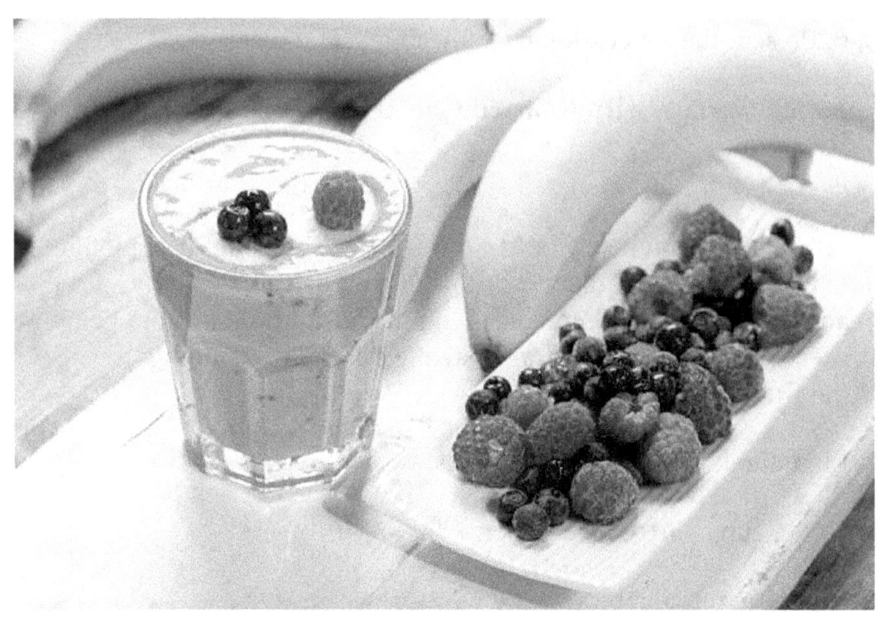

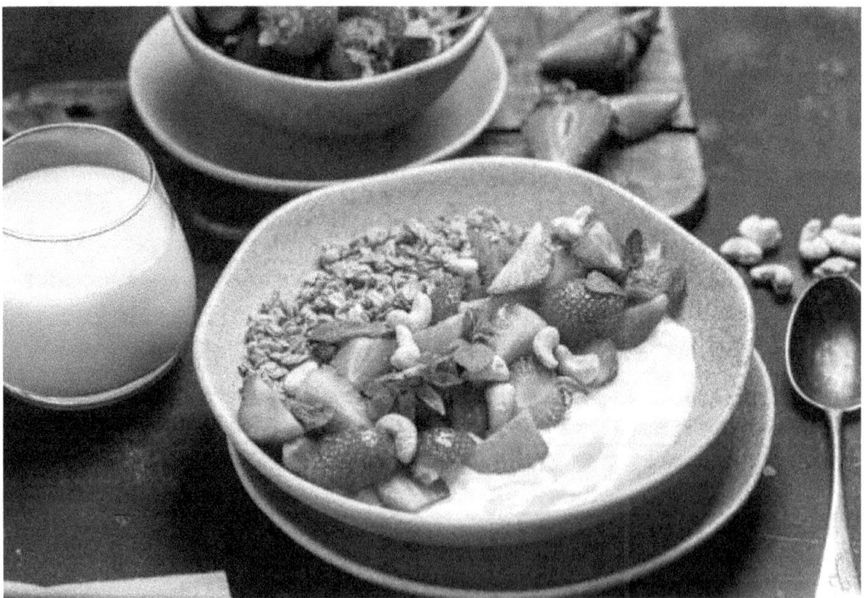

51

Banana, Blueberry, and Strawberry Smoothie 10. Strawberry Muesli

This simple meal wil provide you with complete grains, fiber, and protein to start your day.

Ingredients

⅓ cup granola

One cup of raspberries

1/4 cup nonfat milk

Preparation

Add raspberries to the muesli and serve with milk.

Strawberry Muesli

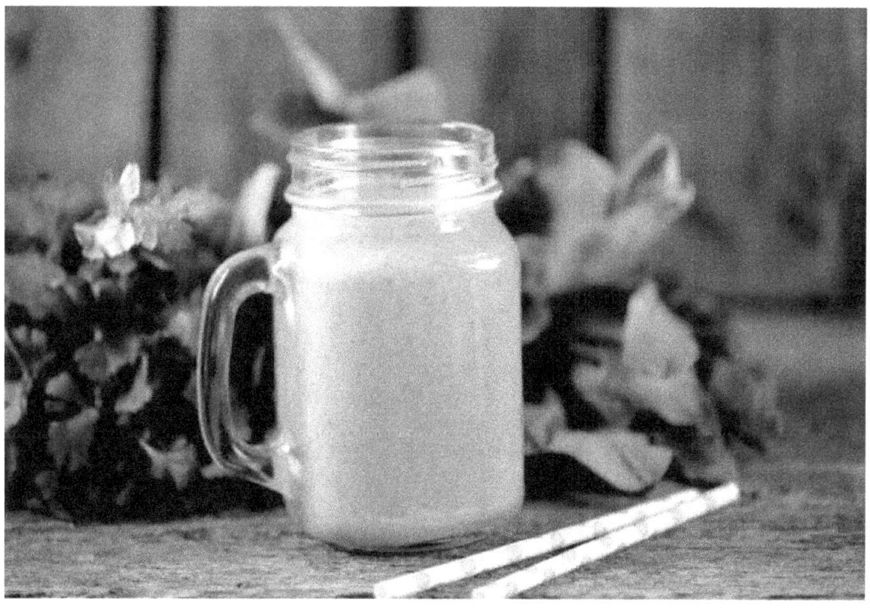

52

Collagen Smoothies

1. Power Green Smoothie

This 5-minute recipe for a strong green smoothie includes al the ingredients you need to look and feel younger! Diminish the indications of age, enhance vitality, and feel equipped to tackle the day!

Ingredients

one cup spinach

one cup kale

1 cup of mango, frozen

1/4 banana

One cup of your preferred almond milk

One scoop of your preferred col agen powder Preparation

Put al items into a large food processor or blender. Mix until homogeneous.

Power Green Smoothie

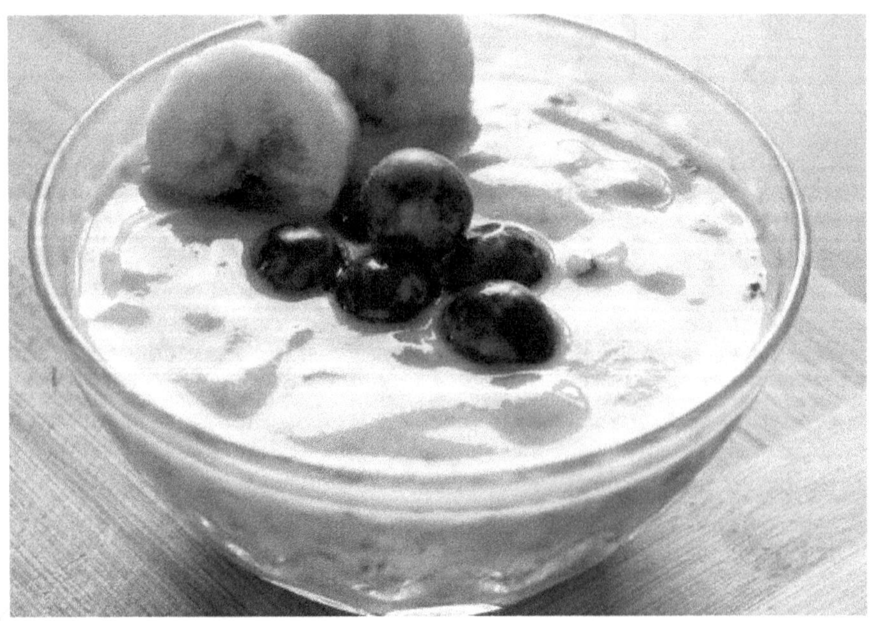

2. Superb Berry Banana Smoothie

With this tasty banana berry smoothie recipe, bid adieu to your foggy morning brain! Your memory and focus are improved by the superfoods in this smoothie, enabling you to tackle the day!

Ingredients

1 frozen ripe banana

1 cup of blueberries, frozen

One container (5.3 ounces) of vanil a Greek yogurt (about 1/2 cup) Almond milk, one cup

two heaping tablespoons of your preferred col agen powder Preparation

Put al items into a large food processor or blender. Mix until homogeneous.

Superb Berry Banana Smoothie

3. Smoothed Almonds

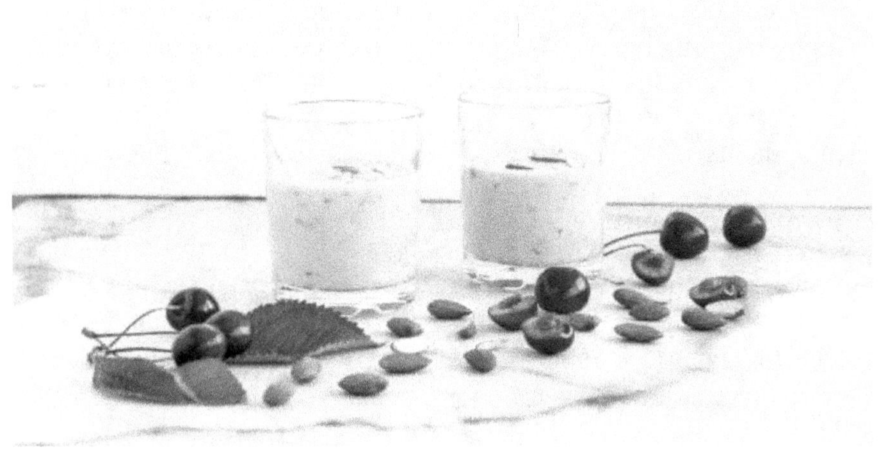

54

This cherry almond smoothie recipe, which cal s for just five ingredients, is incredibly tasty, anti-aging, and ful of healthful antioxidants. You'l be eager to make it again and over again!

Ingredients

One scoop of your preferred col agen powder Pitted 1/2 Cup Cherries

Almonds, 1/4 cup

1 cup plain or vanil a Greek yogurt and 1/2 teaspoon rose water As needed, add almond milk.

Preparation

Put al the ingredients in a blender and process until the mixture is smooth.

Pour into a glass and savor!

Smoothed Almonds

4. Meal Substitute Shake for Luminous Skin

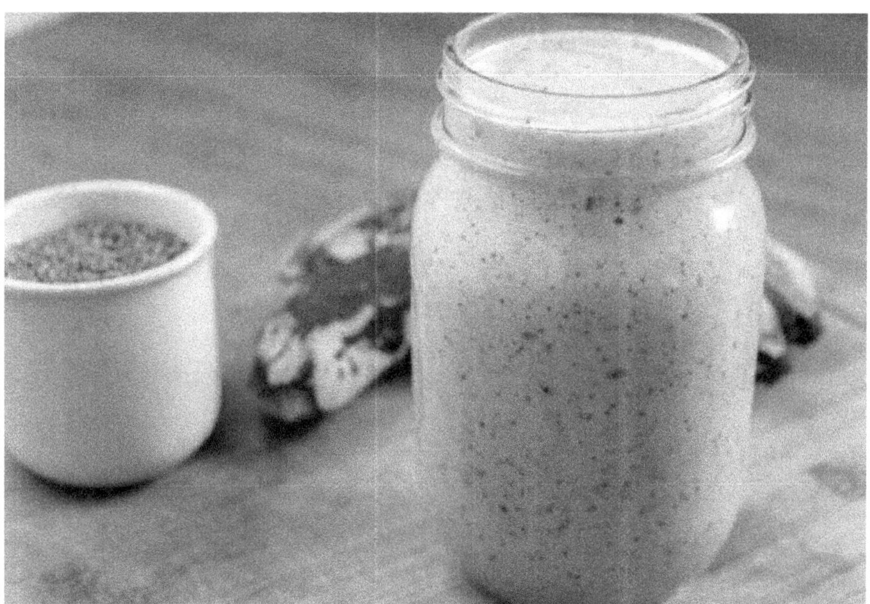

55

Discover how to create a meal replacement smoothie that can aid in weight loss and leave your skin looking radiant and alive! For quick results, try this recipe for a col agen smoothie!

Ingredients

One cup almond milk, or dairy-free milk two heaping tablespoons of your preferred col agen powder 1 cup of spinach

One banana, frozen

One tablespoon of nut butter

One tablespoon ground or whole flaxseed A half-tsp vanil a extract

1 tsp of optional cinnamon ice

Preparation

Place al components in a strong blender and process until smooth.

Meal Substitute Shake for Luminous Skin

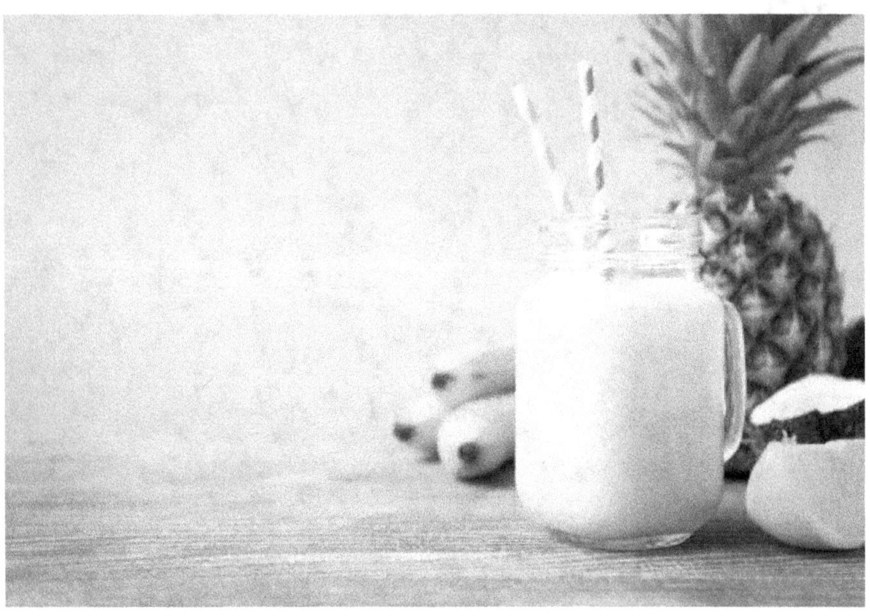

56

5. Nutritious Piña Colada Drink Recipe This healthy piña colada smoothie recipe is perfect for you if you love pina coladas but detest al the added sugar and calories!

Ingredients

One frozen banana, cut.

Two cups of pineapple chunks, frozen or fresh One cup of light vanil a coconut milk

1/4 teaspoon vanil a extract

One or two scoops of your preferred col agen powder Preparation

Using a strong blender, combine frozen bananas, pineapple chunks, coconut milk, vanil a essence, and col agen powder of your choice,process until smooth. Have fun!

Nutritious Piña Colada Drink Recipe

57

Healthy snacks

1. Light Parfait with Pumpkin Pie

This tasty and easy recipe for a light pumpkin pie parfait is perfect for those who enjoy pumpkin pie and whipped cream! Half the calories but the same delicious taste!

Ingredients

14 oz. (one can) pureed pumpkin

two eggs

One-third cup lemon juice

Half a cup almond milk

1/4 cup of pure maple syrup

½ tsp of spice for pumpkin pie

Salt, ½ teaspoon

Two cups of vanil a Greek yogurt without fat two heaping tablespoons of your preferred col agen powder Pecans (as garnishes)

Preparation

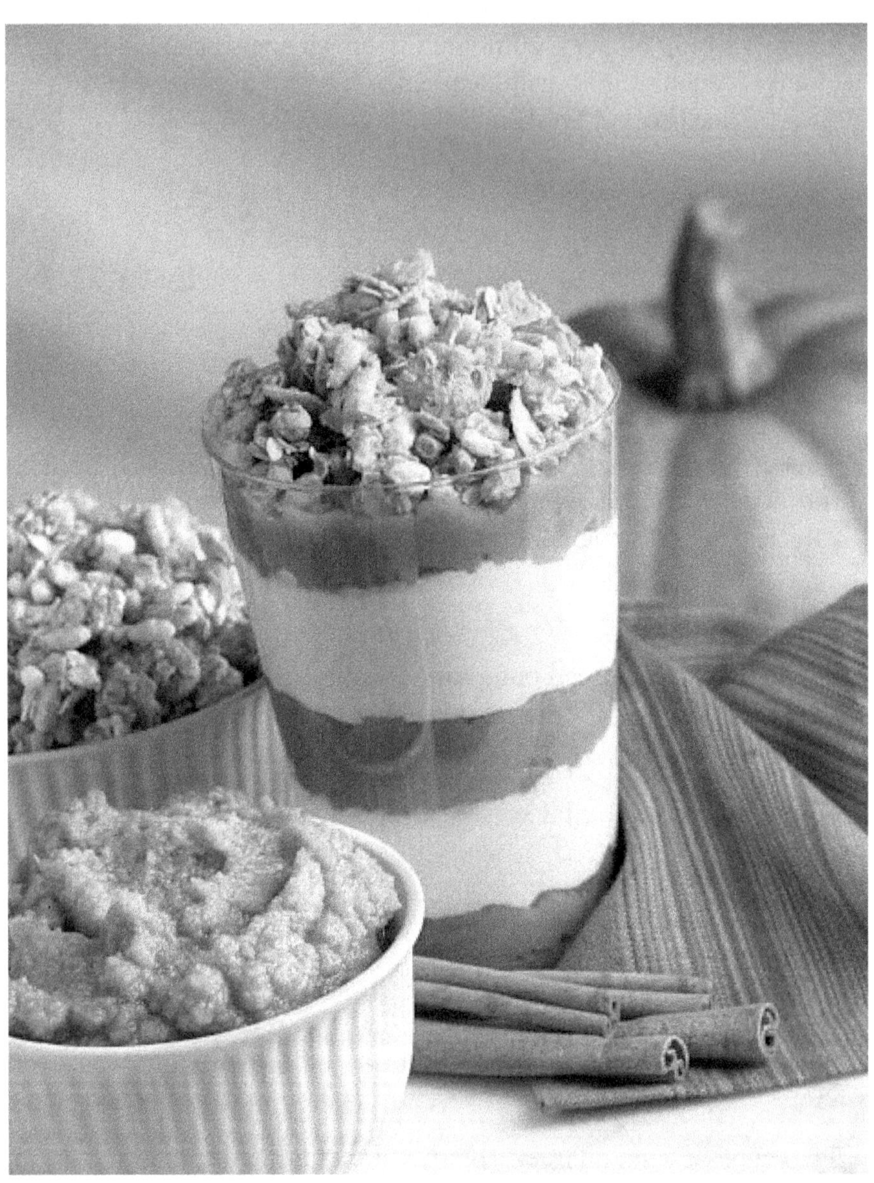

58

1. Set the oven's temperature to 350.

Pumpkin puree, eggs, milk, lemon juice, maple syrup, pumpkin pie spice, and salt should al be combined in a big basin. Mix wel until wel blended.

2. Transfer the blend into a baking dish. For 30 minutes, bake. Al ow the mixture to cool for ten minutes or more after baking.

3. Add your col agen powder to the Greek yogurt and stir until combined while the pumpkin mixture bakes.

4. To assemble the parfaits, fil a smal glass or jar ¼ ful with the pumpkin mixture. Next, cover the pumpkin mixture with ¼ cup of the col agen yogurt.

Yogurt and the pumpkin mixture are layered again.

5. Add extra nuts, maple syrup, and pumpkin spice pecan granola to the top of each parfait, if preferred.

Light Parfait with Pumpkin Pie

2. Nutritional Pumpkin Muffins

59

Enjoy these nutritious pumpkin muffins al year long to feel snug and pleasant fal sensations! Not only do they include an abundance of heart-healthy and fiber nutrients, but they also have no gluten!

Ingredients

3 cups old-fashioned oats* 1 tablespoon spice for pumpkin pie ½ teaspoon baking soda

½ teaspoon fine sea salt

two eggs

Two scoops of your preferred, unflavored col agen powder 1 cup almond milk without sugar

one cup pureed pumpkin

1/4 cup of maple syrup

Three tablespoons of melted coconut oil, or any oil with a mild flavor One teaspoon vanil a extract

Optional add-ins: walnuts or raisins

Sprinkle some Turbinado sugar on top if you'd like.

Preparation

60

1. Turn the oven on to 375°F. Grease a 12-cup muffin pan (or a large 6-cup muffin pan) liberal y with cooking spray, then line with parchment or cupcake liners. Put away.

2. Using a blender or food processor, puree the oats until they resemble flour. Pulse in the baking soda, sea salt, col agen powder, and pumpkin pie spice until the mixture is wel blended. Put away.

3. In a different, sizable mixing basin, thoroughly mix the eggs, almond milk, pureed pumpkin, maple syrup, coconut oil, and vanil a extract. Stir the mixture until it is just incorporated, then fold in the dry ingredients along with the wet ingredient mixture.

4. Spoon mixture into baking cups that have been prepared. If desired, dust the tops with sugar.

5. Bake for 15 to 18 minutes if using a 12-muffin tin. If you're using a large muffin pan with a capacity of 6 cups, bake the muffins for 25 to 28 minutes, or until a toothpick inserted in the center comes out clean. Take the pan out of the oven and let it cool for five minutes on a cooling rack.

6. You can freeze the muffins for up to three months, or serve them warm and al ow them to cool to room temperature before storing them in a tight container.

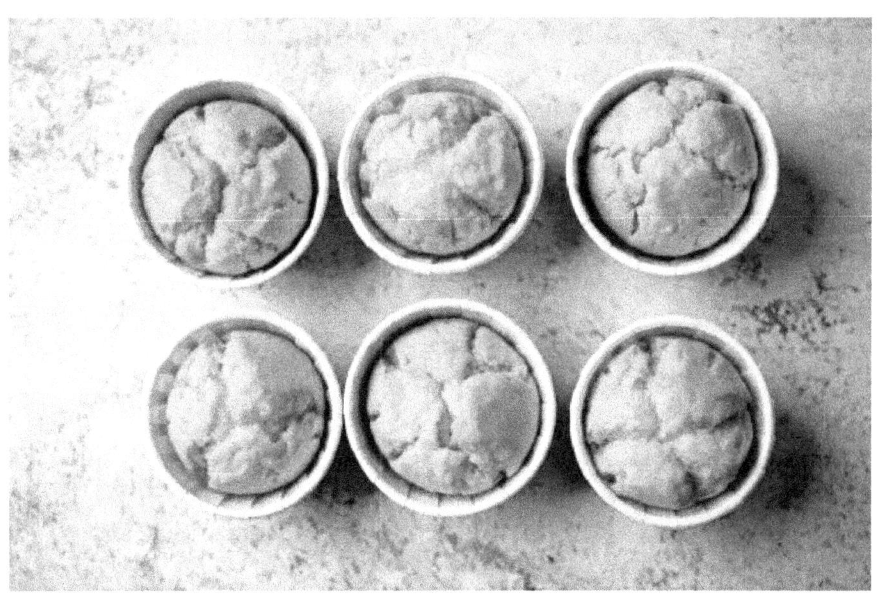

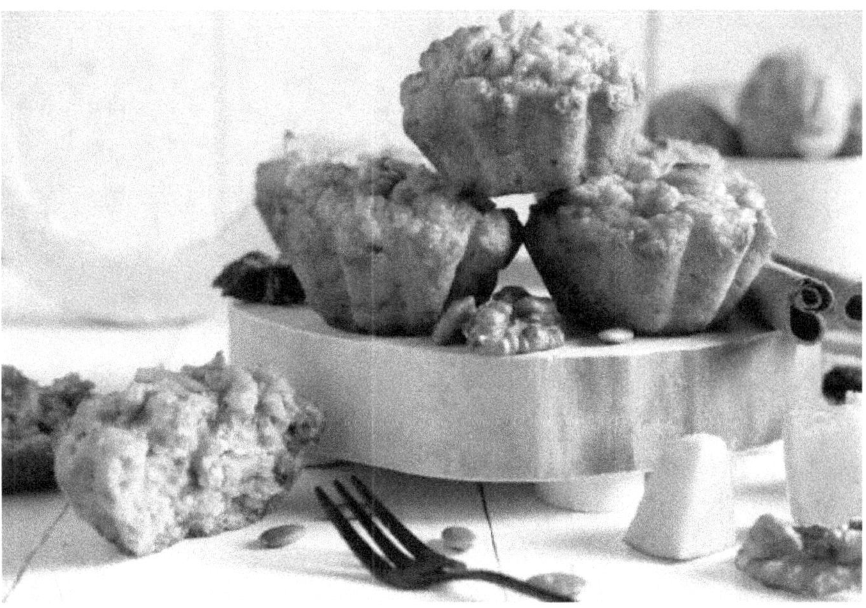

61

Nutritional Pumpkin

Muffins

3. Poppy Seed and Blueberry Lemon Muffins These nutritious blueberry lemon poppyseed muffins are the ideal way to start the day! Rich in protein, soluble fiber, and our top-secret, age-defying ingredient!

Ingredients

Two big eggs

¼ cup of plain Greek yogurt at 2%

Two medium-sized, ripe bananas (about one cup), mashed ½ cup brown sugar OR coconut palm sugar, depending on what's most convenient.

One teaspoon vanil a extract

One teaspoon of baking soda

1/4 teaspoon ground cinnamon

½ cup of quick oats

62

Cup of oat flour

two tablespoons of your preferred col agen powder One cup of fresh or frozen blueberries

One to two tablespoons of lemon zest, depending on desired level of zing Tbsp of poppy seeds

Preparation

1. Set aside a muffin tin and preheat the oven to 350ºF. Line the cavities with parchment paper liners or coat the pan with cooking spray. Put away.

2. Lightly whisk the eggs in a large mixing bowl until the yolks separate.

Add the yogurt, bananas, vanil a, and zest of the lemon and blend until smooth. Stir in sugar thoroughly.

3. Combine the col agen powder, flour, oats, baking soda, and cinnamon in another bowl, and wel mix.

4. Spoon in flour mixture; whisk in poppyseeds gently until wel incorporated. Fold the blueberries into the batter after tossing them in 1

Tbsp flour to stop them from leaking or sinking to the bottom of the muffins.

5. Evenly distribute the batter among the 12 muffin cups, fil ing them nearly to the brim. If preferred, top with a sprinkling of coconut sugar.

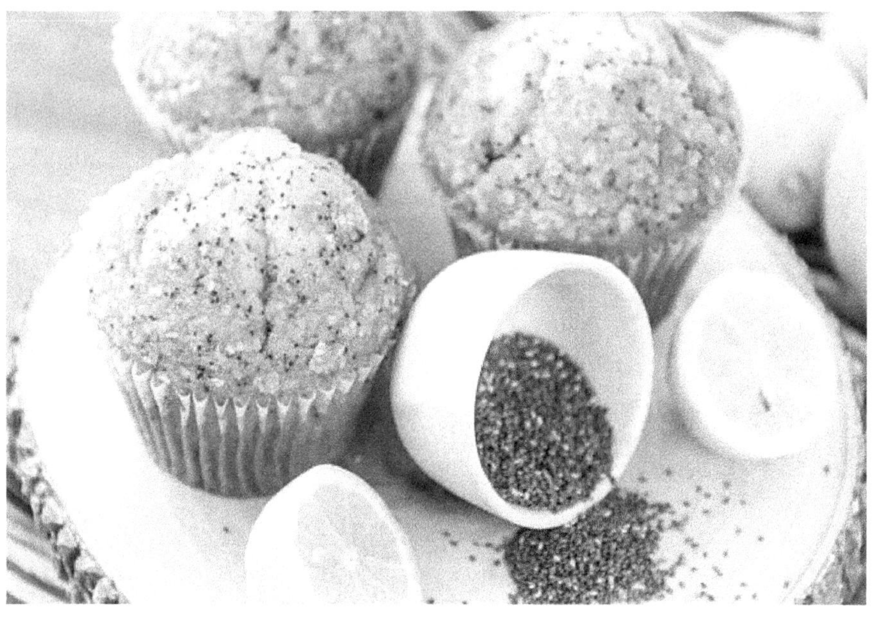

63

6. Bake for 20 to 22 minutes, or until a toothpick inserted into the center of the muffins comes out clean and the tops of the muffins start to turn golden brown. After letting the muffins cool in the pan

for about five minutes, move them to a wire rack to finish cooling. You can freeze them for up to three months, or keep them at room temperature for up to five days in an airtight container.

Poppy Seed and Blueberry Lemon Muffins 4. Strawberry Jam Made at Home

Try this 4-ingredient homemade strawberry jam recipe if you're looking for a healthy jam that doesn't have a lot of added sugar or calories! You won't believe what our secret ingredient is!

Ingredients

Two cups of pure strawberry

Two tablespoons of chia seeds

1/4 cup of honey.

two tablespoons of your preferred col agen powder

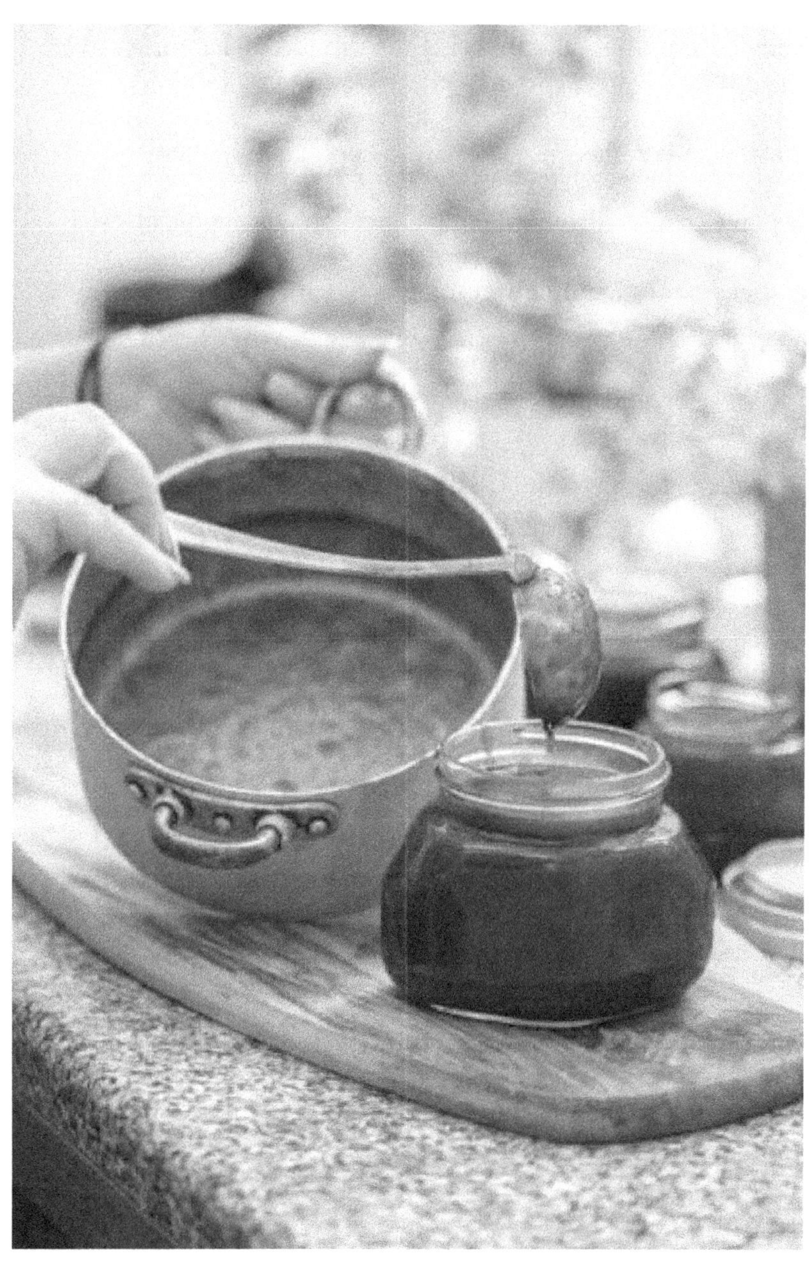

64

Preparation

1. Use a blender to puree al items for 30 seconds.

2. Transfer to a smal pot and bring the mixture to a simmer over low heat.

3. Transfer into a glass jar, al ow it to cool, and refrigerate.

4. Use on Col agen Protein Donuts or on breads and pastries!

Strawberry Jam Made at Home

5. Acai Bowl

Ingredients

One generous spoonful of your preferred col agen powder One banana, frozen

One cup of mixed frozen berries

One tablespoon honey

One packet of frozen acai, broken into pieces ⅓ cup almond milk (more may be required to achieve the desired consistency).

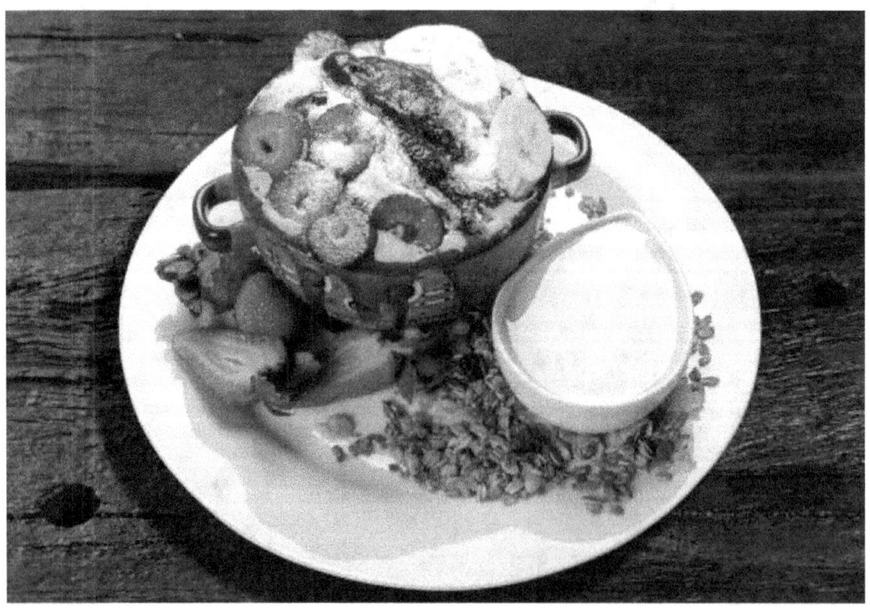

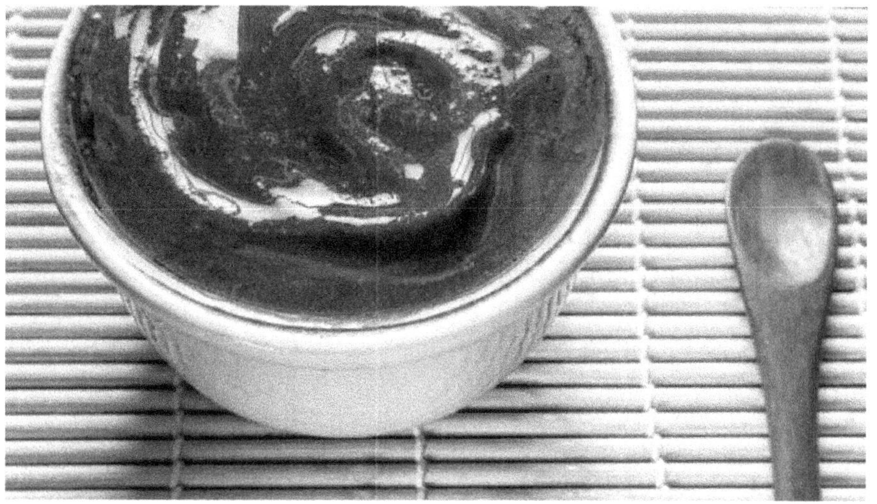

65

* Strong blender

Preparation

1. Fil the blender with the frozen berries, banana, almond milk, col agen powder, honey, and acai pieces.

2. Blend until wel incorporated; you might need to add extra almond milk if the mixture is too clumpy. The finished mixture ought to be thick and smooth, not clumpy or watery.)

3. Transfer the smoothie mixture to a bowl and top with your preferred ingredients. Serve right away.

Acai Bowl

Extra Toppings

1.Coconut flakes, strawberry, and kiwi in a glowing bowl
2.Granola, blueberries, and fresh banana slices for an energy boost
3.Flaxseed, strawberries, blackberries, and blueberries are super antioxidants.

66

4.Nourishing Brain: Almonds, Pumpkin Seeds, Raspberries
5.Chocolate Addiction: Dark cherries, coconut flakes, strawberries, and cocoa nibs

Conclusion

You have read about the advantages of col agen for women's wel ness, appearance, and health in this book. You've also learned how to improve your col agen intake with food, supplements, and way of life adjustments.

You may enhance your skin, hair, nails, joints, bones, muscles, intestines, and immune system by adhering to the col agen diet for women.

Additional y, you can stop or even cure age-related symptoms like wrinkles,

67

sagging skin, dryness, and inflammation. In addition to being a protein, col agen is an extremely effective al y for your general health. I hope you found this book to be enjoyable, insightful, and motivating to read. Keep in mind that col agen can enhance your natural beauty. You are already stunning on the inside and out.